THE *Skinny*
SPIRALIZER
SOUP
RECIPE BOOK

 CookNation

THE SKINNY SPIRALIZER SOUP RECIPE BOOK

Delicious Spiralizer Inspired Soup Recipes All
Under 100, 200, 300 & 400 Calories

ISBN 978-1-909855-92-2

A CIP catalogue record of this book is available from the
British Library

CONTENTS

UNDER 300 CALORIES

UNDER 400 CALORIES

INTRODUCTION

"Good soup is one of the prime ingredients of good living. For soup can do more to lift the spirits and stimulate the appetite than any other one dish."

Louis P. De Gouy, 'The Soup Book' (1949)

Soup is the ultimate comfort food: warm, hearty, filling, tasty, healthy and easy to make. It comes in a multitude of different forms: creamy, textured, chunky, hot or cold, spicy, tangy... the list goes on. Made from fresh ingredients or leftover cuts from the kitchen, soup can find a place in every kitchen.

Our skinny soups are balanced, healthy low calorie, delicious and now thanks to a vegetable spiralizer can be even more fun to make and eat.

The joy of using a vegetable spiralizer to create fun veggie noodles, spaghetti, ribbons, 'rice', spirals and more can take your soups to a whole new level.

The vegetable spiralizer isn't just for vegetarians. Our skinny soups include, meat, seafood and vegetables options and are perfect as part of a balanced diet. They can be instrumental in helping you lose weight or maintain your figure without compromising on flavour, taste or leaving you feeling hungry. All our recipes serve 4 and fall under either 100, 200, 300 or 400 calories per serving.

You don't have to be a great chef to make a great soup. All our skinny spiralizer soups are easy to make with readily sourced ingredients and minimum prep time.

These are the key elements to making a great soup:

THE BASE
Most soups require a few vegetables to give your soup a rounded flavour. Onions, carrots and celery are a great place to start.

STOCK
A good quality stock will make the world of difference to the taste of your soup. Use either vegetable, fish or meat stock and if you can make these at home, all the better. You can follow these simple instructions to make homemade stock. If you opt for store-bought stock try to choose a good quality product that is not high in sodium.

INGREDIENTS

Soup is so versatile that almost any ingredient can be used whether you are looking for a meaty protein packed dish, an Asian seafood soup, or a thick vegetarian broth using beans and pulses. Certain ingredients will change the consistency of your soup too, for example potatoes and lentils will thicken, while adding cream or yogurt will make it smoother.

SEASONING

Most soups will require some seasoning. Be careful when choosing your stock that it is not overly high in its sodium content. There are also many popular herbs that compliment soups such as marjoram, thyme, parsley, sage, rosemary, oregano and of course salt and pepper. You should also feel free to experiment. For example: Garlic, ginger and coriander can work well in Asian soups while cumin, turmeric or garam masala can give an authentic Indian feel to your soup.

GARNISH

There is nothing better than serving a homemade soup with a little garnish, which not only looks the part but also adds an extra taste. Depending on your dish, freshly chopped herbs, croutons, a little cream, crème fraiche or freshly grated parmesan are all great finishing touches. We have also included a garnish section which should give you some new ideas too.

OUR SKINNY RECIPES

All the recipes in this book are a guide only. You may need to alter quantities and cooking times to suit your own cooking equipment.

Consistency is also a question of personal preference. Some recipes suggest the best consistency to use; others leave it to your own personal taste. Feel free to experiment by adding more or less stock to suit your own taste.

All our recipes are simple and easy to follow and all fall below 100, 200, 300 or 400 calories each. Many use low calorie and low fat alternatives to everyday products. We would encourage you to add these to your shopping basket each week and make a point of paying attention to food labelling whenever you can - some low fat products can be very high in sugar so watch out! Try switching to some of the following everyday items to keep calories and fat lower:

Low fat yogurt
Semi skimmed/ half fat milk
Reduced fat cheese
Low fat/unsaturated 'butter' spreads
Low cal cooking oil spray
Low fat cream/ half and half

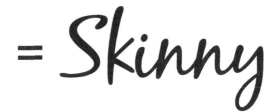

ABOUT SPIRALIZING

In its most basic form, a spiralizer turns vegetables into noodles – a godsend for anyone who loves pasta – but can also create veggie spaghetti, ribbons, spirals and more, making vegetables at mealtimes an art form. It is a manual gadget that requires no electricity. Gripping a vegetable like a vice and cranking the handle pushes the vegetable through a sharp blade to create vegetable spirals. Once spiralized, you are left with the central core of the vegetable which can either be discarded or chopped up and used in your recipe – great for soups!

The most popular spiralizer devices come with 3 interchangeable blades. The names of these blades may differ depending on which device you own but they will all deliver similar results:

• •

Shredder Blade – creates thin spaghetti-like noodles
Chipper Blade – creates thicker noodles
Straight/Slicer Blade – creates ribbons/slices

• •

The blades are very sharp and care should be taken when handling and cleaning them. It helps to use a knife to remove any leftover vegetable from the blades before washing.

The spiralizer comes with rubber suction cups on the base that provide much needed stability when applying pressure to turn the handle. Push the device down firmly on your counter top to prevent sliding and have a bowl/plate/chopping board in place to catch the spirals.

Cleaning your spiralizer couldn't be easier. It should come apart into 3 main components: the base, the handle and the blade. Everything except the metal blade is made of plastic which can be easily washed or placed in the dishwasher (blades included). Just make sure you rinse everything under the tap first to remove any leftover vegetable.

There are a number of vegetables that work particularly well with the spiralizer. Some won't work so well. Generally speaking vegetables that are hollow, are too small or don't have a solid shape are not suitable for spiralizing. Remember that while there are plenty of vegetables that may not be suitable for spiralizing, they can still be added to your soup. Most of our recipes use a wide range of veg to make up your meal.

When shopping for your vegetables try to choose larger, fatter varieties as they give much better results.

The emphasis of this recipe book is healthy, low calorie soups so it's important to remember not to use excessive amounts of cooking oil that can be high in saturated fats and calories. Make sure you have to hand a good quality extra virgin olive oil and low calorie cooking oil spray. Only a small amount is needed to cook evenly. Using good quality non-stick pans will also reduce the need for excessive oil.

We hope you enjoy using your spiralizer to create wonderful homemade soups and draw inspiration to craft your own delicious dishes.

ABOUT COOKNATION

CookNation is the leading publisher of innovative and practical recipe books for the modern, health-conscious cook.

CookNation titles bring together delicious, easy and practical recipes with their unique approach - making cooking for diets and healthy eating fast, simple and fun.

With a range of #1 best-selling titles - from the innovative 'Skinny' calorie-counted series, to the 5:2 Diet Recipes Collection - CookNation recipe books prove that 'Diet' can still mean 'Delicious'!

Browse our catalogue by searching under **'CookNation'** on Amazon or visit **www.cooknationbooks.com** and **www.bellmackenzie.com**

Skinny
SPIRALIZER
SOUPS

UNDER 100 CALORIES

SPINACH RAMEN

95
calories per
serving

Ingredients

- 600g/1lb 5oz courgettes/zucchini
- 200g/7oz carrots
- 200g/7oz mushroom, thinly sliced
- 200g/7oz spinach, roughly chopped
- 3 tbsp miso paste
- 1.5lt/6 cups boiling water
- 2 tbsp soy sauce
- Salt & pepper to taste

Method

1 Top & tail the courgettes and use the shredder blade to turn into thin noodles.

2 Do the same with the carrots, peeling them first.

3 Add everything, except the soy sauce, to a large non-stick saucepan on the hob and gently simmer for 5 minutes or until the carrots & courgettes are tender.

4 Season and serve with the soy sauce dashed over the top of each bowl.

CHEFS NOTE

Try garnishing the soup with a handful of finely sliced spring onions.

COURGETTE & CARROT MISO SOUP

80 calories per serving

Ingredients

- 600g/1lb 5oz courgettes/zucchini
- 200g/7oz carrots
- 3 tbsp miso paste
- 1.25lt/5 cups boiling water
- Salt & pepper to taste

Method

1 Top & tail the courgettes and use the shredder blade to turn into thin noodles.

2 Do the same with the carrots, peeling them first.

3 Add everything to a large non-stick saucepan on the hob and gently simmer for 5 minutes or until the carrots & courgettes are tender.

4 Season and serve.

CHEFS NOTE

This is a really simple miso soup. Adjust the quantity of paste to suit your own taste.

GREEN TEA & VEGGIE MISO SOUP

85
calories per serving

Ingredients

- 2 green tea bags
- 1.25lt/5 cups boiling water
- 600g/1lb 5oz courgettes/zucchini
- 200g/7oz carrots
- ½ tsp ground ginger

- 3 tbsp miso paste
- 2 tbsp soy sauce
- Large bunch spring onions, finely chopped
- Salt & pepper to taste

Method

1 Place the teabags in the boiling water and leave for a few minutes whilst you prepare the vegetables.

2 Top & tail the courgettes and use the shredder blade to turn into thin noodles. Do the same with the carrots, peeling them first.

3 Heat a large non-stick saucepan on the hob and add the green tea water (remove the teabags first). Stir through the ginger, miso paste & soy sauce and simmer for a minute or two until these have dissolved into the soup base.

4 Add the carrot and courgette noodles and gently simmer for 3-4 minutes or until everything is tender & piping hot.

5 Season and serve with the spring onions sprinkled over the top.

CHEFS NOTE

This is a really simple miso soup. Adjust the quantity of paste to suit your own taste.

NO-COOK CUCUMBER SOUP

80 calories per serving

Ingredients

- 4 cucumbers
- 1 tbsp each freshly chopped basil & dill
- 750ml/3 cups cooled vegetable stock
- 250ml/1 cup fat free Greek yogurt
- 1 tsp paprika
- Salt & pepper to taste

Method

1 Place 3 of the cucumbers along with the chopped herbs, cooled vegetable stock and yogurt in a blender. Blend until smooth.

2 Meanwhile top & tail the remaining cucumber and use the shredder blade to turn into thin noodles.

3 Divide the chilled soup into bowl and sit a mound of cucumber noodles on top. Sprinkle with paprika and serve.

CHEFS NOTE
This simple chilled soup is really refreshing on a hot day.

Skinny
SPIRALIZER
SOUPS

UNDER 200 CALORIES

PAK CHOI & CHILLI SOUP

145
calories per serving

Ingredients

- 600g/1lb 5oz courgettes/zucchini
- 1 tbsp olive oil
- 1 onion, finely chopped
- 1 tsp freshly grated ginger
- 2 red chillies, deseeded & finely chopped
- 1 garlic clove, crushed

- 1.5l/6 cups chicken or vegetable stock
- 200g/7oz potatoes, peeled & cubed
- 2 pak choi, shredded
- 2 tsp brown sugar
- Salt & pepper to taste

Method

1 Top & tail the courgettes and use the shredder blade to turn into thin spirals.

2 Take a knife and, holding the spirals in bunches, roughly chop into 1cm/½ inch pieces.

3 Gently heat a large non-stick saucepan on the hob with the olive oil and sauté the onions, ginger, chillies & garlic for 5 minutes until softened.

4 Add the stock, potatoes & sugar and cook for 6-8 minutes or until the potatoes are tender.

5 Tip the contents of the pan into a blender and blend until smooth.

6 Return to the pan with the courgettes & pak choi. Cover and simmer for 3-5 minutes or everything is tender and the soup is piping hot.

7 Season and serve.

CHEFS NOTE

Shredded white cabbage will work in place of pak choi.

BROCCOLI & HORSERADISH SOUP

195 calories per serving

Ingredients

- 600g/1lb 5oz courgettes/zucchini
- 1 tbsp olive oil
- 1 onion, finely chopped
- 3 garlic cloves, crushed
- 200g/7oz potatoes, peeled & cubed
- 1.5l/6 cups chicken or vegetable stock
- 2 tbsp horseradish sauce
- 150g/5oz purple sprouting broccoli/broccolini, finely chopped
- Zest of one lime
- Salt & pepper to taste

Method

1 Top & tail the courgettes and use the shredder blade to turn into thin noodles.

2 Gently heat a large non-stick saucepan on the hob with the olive oil and sauté the onions, garlic & potatoes for a few minutes until softened.

3 Add the stock and horseradish sauce and cook for 6-8 minutes or until the potatoes are tender.

4 Tip the contents of the pan into a blender and blend until smooth. Return to the pan with the chopped broccoli and courgette noodles. Cover and simmer for 3-5 minutes or until everything is tender and the soup is piping hot.

5 Season and serve with the lime zest sprinkled over the top.

CHEFS NOTE
Alter the quantity of horseradish to suit your own taste.

SWEET TOMATO & 'RICE' SOUP

185
calories per serving

Ingredients

- 400g/14oz sweet potatoes
- 1 tbsp olive oil
- 1 onion, finely chopped
- 1 carrot, finely chopped
- 1 tbsp brown sugar
- 2 tbsp balsamic vinegar

- 1 tbsp tomato puree
- 500ml/2 cups tomato passata/sieved tomatoes
- 1lt/4 cups vegetable or chicken stock
- Salt & pepper to taste

Method

1 Peel the sweet potatoes and use the chipper blade to turn into thick spirals.

2 Take a knife and, holding the spirals in bunches, roughly chop into 1cm/½ inch pieces.

3 Heat a large non-stick saucepan on the hob with the olive oil and gently sauté the onions & carrots for a few minutes until softened. Stir though the sugar, vinegar and puree and cook for a little longer until the sugar dissolves.

4 Add the passata, stock & chopped sweet potato and simmer for 5-8 minutes or until the sweet potato is tender and the soup is piping hot.

5 Check the seasoning and serve.

CHEFS NOTE

Use tinned chopped tomatoes in place of passata if you prefer.

CREAMY PARSLEY SOUP

175 calories per serving

Ingredients

- 400g/14oz courgettes/zucchini
- 1 tbsp olive oil
- 1 onion, chopped
- 1 garlic clove, crushed
- 400g/14oz potatoes, peeled & diced
- Large bunch of fresh parsley (remove the thickest stalks)
- 1.25lt/5 cups chicken or vegetable stock
- Salt & pepper to taste

Method

1 Top & tail the courgettes and use the chipper blade to turn into thick spirals.

2 Take a knife and, holding the spirals in bunches, roughly chop into 1cm/½ inch pieces.

3 Heat a large non-stick saucepan on the hob with the olive oil and gently sauté the onions, garlic & potatoes for a few minutes until softened. Add the parsley & stock and cook for a 5-7 minutes until the potatoes are tender.

4 Tip the contents of the saucepan into a blender and pulse until smooth.

5 Return the soup to the pan along with the chopped courgette and simmer for 3-4 minutes or until the chopped courgette is tender and the soup is piping hot.

6 Season and serve.

CHEFS NOTE
Reserve a little of the fresh parsley for garnishing.

BASIL & COURGETTE RIBBON SOUP

165
calories per serving

Ingredients

- 800g/1¾lb courgettes/zucchini
- 1 tbsp olive oil
- 1 onion, chopped
- 2 garlic cloves, crushed
- 2 tbsp tomato puree/paste

- 4 tbsp freshly chopped basil
- 1lt/3 cups chicken or vegetable stock
- 400g/14oz tinned chopped tomatoes
- 4 tbsp fat free Greek yogurt
- Salt & pepper to taste

Method

1 Top & tail the courgettes and use the straight/slicer blade to turn into thick ribbons.

2 Gently heat a large non-stick saucepan on the hob with the olive oil. Add the chopped onions & garlic and gently sauté for a few minutes until softened.

3 Stir through the puree and add the fresh basil, stock, ribbons & chopped tomatoes. Cover and leave to simmer for 3-4 minutes or until everything is tender and piping hot.

4 Season and serve the soup in shallow bowls with a dollop of Greek yogurt in the centre of each.

CHEFS NOTE
Reserve a little of the fresh basil or use extra as a garnish.

SQUASH 'RICE' & SPICED TOMATO SOUP

175
calories per serving

Ingredients

- 800g/1¾lb butternut squash
- 1 tbsp olive oil
- 2 garlic cloves, crushed
- 1 onion, finely chopped
- 1 carrot, finely chopped
- 1 tsp ground cumin & coriander/cilantro
- 400g/14oz tinned chopped tomatoes
- 1.25lt/5 cups vegetable or chicken stock
- Salt & pepper to taste

Method

1 Peel the squash and use the chipper blade to turn into thick spirals.

2 Take a knife and, holding the spirals in bunches, roughly chop into 1cm/½ inch pieces.

3 Heat a large non-stick saucepan on the hob with the olive oil and gently sauté the onions & carrots for a few minutes until softened. Stir though the dried spices, add the tomatoes, stock & squash and simmer for 5-7 minutes or until the sweet potatoes are tender and the soup is piping hot.

4 Check the seasoning and serve.

CHEFS NOTE
Add some dried chilli flakes to this simple soup if you want some 'heat'.

SQUASH SPIRAL & FLAGEOLET SOUP

195 calories per serving

Ingredients

- 600g/1lb 5oz butternut squash
- 1 onion, chopped
- 1 tbsp olive oil
- 2 celery stalks, chopped
- 2 garlic cloves, crushed
- 2 tsp dried mixed herbs
- 300g/11oz tinned flageolet beans
- 200g/7oz spinach
- 1.25lt/5 cups chicken or vegetable stock
- Salt & pepper to taste

Method

1 Peel the squash and use the chipper blade to turn into thick spirals.

2 Gently heat a large non-stick saucepan pan on the hob with the olive oil. Add the chopped onions, celery & garlic and gently sauté for a few minutes until softened.

3 Stir through the mixed herbs. Add the beans, spinach, stock & squash spirals and cook for 8-10 minutes or until the spirals are tender and the soup is piping hot.

4 Check the seasoning and serve.

CHEFS NOTE

Chose a long stemmed squash shape as you won't be able to spiralize the 'bulb' end where all the seeds are.

TURNIP & KALE, BEAN SOUP

190 calories per serving

Ingredients

- 800g/1¾lb turnip
- 1 onion, chopped
- 1 tbsp olive oil
- 2 garlic cloves, crushed
- 2 tbsp tomato puree/paste
- 1 tsp dried thyme
- 300g/11oz tinned cannellini beans
- 200g/7oz kale
- 1.25lt/5 cups chicken or vegetable stock
- 200g/7oz tinned chopped tomatoes
- Salt & pepper to taste

Method

1 Peel the turnip and use the chipper blade to turn into thick spirals.

2 Gently heat a large non-stick frying pan on the hob with the olive oil. Add the chopped onions & garlic and gently sauté for a few minutes until softened.

3 Stir through the puree and thyme. Add the beans, kale, stock & chopped tomatoes and cook for 2 minutes.

4 Add the turnip spirals and cook for 8-10 minutes or until the spirals are tender and the soup is piping hot.

5 Check the seasoning and serve.

CHEFS NOTE

Turnip is not the easiest vegetable to spiralize. Try choosing a longer more pointed shape if you can, or substitute for sweet potato if you prefer.

MUSHROOM RAMEN

135
calories per
serving

Ingredients

- 800g/1¾lb courgettes/zucchini
- 1 tbsp olive oil
- 1 onion, sliced
- 300g/11oz oyster mushrooms, finely sliced
- 2 pak choi/bok choi, shredded
- 1 tsp crushed chilli flakes
- 1.5lt/6 cups chicken or vegetable stock
- Salt & pepper to taste

Method

1 Top & tail the courgettes and use the shredder blade to turn into thin noodles.

2 Gently heat a large non-stick saucepan on the hob with the olive oil and sauté the sliced onions & mushrooms for 10 minutes or until softened.

3 Add the pak choi, chilli flakes, stock & noodles and simmer for 3-5 minutes or until the noodles are tender and cooked through.

4 Season and serve.

CHEFS NOTE

Chinese oyster mushrooms are good but any mushrooms will work fine.

BROCCOLI & ANCHOVY 'NOODLE' SOUP

120 calories per serving

Ingredients

- 800g/1¾lb courgettes/zucchini
- 1 tbsp olive oil
- 1 onion, finely chopped
- 3 garlic cloves, crushed
- 150g/5oz purple sprouting broccoli/broccolini, finely chopped
- 1 tbsp anchovy paste
- 1.5l/6 cups chicken or vegetable stock
- Salt & pepper to taste

Method

1 Top & tail the courgettes and use the shredder blade to turn into thin noodles.

2 Gently heat a large non-stick saucepan on the hob with the olive oil and sauté the onions, garlic & broccoli for 5 minutes until softened.

3 Stir through the anchovy paste, add the stock & noodles and simmer for 5 minutes or until the noodles are tender.

4 Season and serve.

CHEFS NOTE
Leave your broccoli stems intact if you prefer.

TRICOLOUR VEGGIE SOUP

190
calories per
serving

Ingredients

- 400g/7oz courgettes/zucchini
- 400g/7oz carrots
- 1 tbsp olive oil
- 1 onion, chopped
- 2 garlic cloves, crushed

- 1 tbsp mixed dried French herbs
- 400g/7oz sweet potatoes, peeled & cubed
- 1.5l/6 cups chicken or vegetable stock
- Salt & pepper to taste

Method

1 Top & tail the courgettes & carrots. Peel the carrots and use the shredder blade to turn both vegetables into thin spirals.

2 Take a knife and, holding the spirals in bunches, roughly chop into 2cm/1 inch pieces.

3 Gently heat a large non-stick saucepan on the hob with the olive oil and sauté the chopped onions, garlic, dried herbs & sweet potatoes for a few minutes until softened. Add the stock and cook for 5-7 minutes or until the sweet potatoes are tender.

4 Place in a blender for a few seconds and blend until smooth.

5 Return to the pan along with the chopped spiral veggies and simmer for 5-7 minutes or until the spirals are tender and the soup is piping hot.

6 Season and serve.

CHEFS NOTE

Whizzing the soup before adding the vegetable spirals will give the soup a thicker base.

DROP EGG 'NOODLE' SOUP

190 calories per serving

Ingredients

- 600g/1lb 5oz courgettes/zucchini
- 1 tbsp olive oil
- 2 garlic cloves, crushed
- 1 large bunch spring onions/scallions, thickly chopped

- 2 pak choi/bok choi, shredded
- 1 tbsp soy sauce
- 1.5l/6 cups chicken or vegetable stock
- 4 free range eggs
- Salt & pepper to taste

Method

1 Top & tail the courgettes and use the shredder blade to turn into thin noodles.

2 Gently heat a large saucepan on the hob with the olive oil and sauté the garlic, spring onions & shredded pak choi for a few minutes until softened.

3 Add the soy sauce & stock and simmer for a minute or two.

4 Beat the eggs in a bowl with a little salt and, whilst stirring the soup, slowly pour the eggs into the saucepan so that they set into long 'strands'.

5 Add the courgette noodles and gently simmer for 2 minutes.

6 Check the seasoning and serve in a shallow bowls.

CHEFS NOTE

Cook the 'noodles' for a little longer if you want them very soft.

SAVOURY MISO SOUP

125
calories per
serving

Ingredients

- 800g/1¾lb courgettes/zucchini
- 1 tbsp olive oil
- 3 celery stalks, chopped
- 2 onions, sliced
- 2 garlic cloves, crushed

- 2 tbsp soy sauce
- 2 tbsp miso paste
- 1lt/4 cups boiling water
- Salt & pepper to taste

Method

1 Top & tail the courgettes and use the shredder blade to turn into thin noodles.

2 Gently heat a large non-stick saucepan on the hob with the olive oil and sauté the sliced celery, onion & garlic for 5 minutes or until softened.

3 Add the soy sauce, miso paste, water & courgette noodles and simmer for 3-5 minutes or until the noodles are tender and cooked through.

CHEFS NOTE
Feel free to add some extra water to stretch the soup a little further if you like.

CRÈME FRAICHE BEETROOT & CARROT SOUP

150 calories per serving

Ingredients

- 400g/14oz beetroot
- 400g/14oz carrots
- 1 tbsp olive oil
- 1 onion, sliced
- 2 garlic cloves, crushed
- 1lt/4 cups vegetable or chicken stock
- 4 tbsp fat free crème fraiche
- Salt & pepper to taste

Method

1 Peel each beetroot and use the shredder blade to turn into thin spirals.

2 Take a knife and, holding the spirals in bunches, roughly chop into 2cm/1 inch pieces.

3 Repeat the process with the carrots (peel, top & tail them first).

4 Gently heat a large non-stick saucepan on the hob with the olive oil and sauté the sliced onion & garlic for 5-7 minutes until softened.

5 Add the stock, beetroot & carrots to the pan and simmer for 8 minutes or until the vegetables are tender and the soup is piping hot.

6 Season, and serve with a dollop of crème fraiche in the centre.

CHEFS NOTE

Try some freshly chopped chives on top of the crème fraiche.

SUGAR SNAP & SWEETCORN BROTH

165 calories per serving

Ingredients

- 800g/1¾lb courgettes/zucchini
- 1 tbsp olive oil
- 2 onions, sliced
- 2 garlic cloves, crushed
- 300g/11oz sugar snap peas
- 200g/7oz tinned sweetcorn
- 1.5l/6 cups vegetable or chicken stock
- Salt & pepper to taste

Method

1 Top & tail the courgettes and use the shredder blade to turn into thin noodles.

2 Gently heat a large non-stick saucepan on the hob with the olive oil and sauté the onions & garlic for 3-5 minutes until softened.

3 Add the peas, sweetcorn, stock & courgette noodles and simmer for 3-5 minutes or until the noodles are tender.

4 Season with plenty of black pepper and serve.

CHEFS NOTE

You could also try making with some tinned, creamed sweetcorn if you want to give this clear broth a thicker 'base'.

SPICY PRAWN BROTH

175 calories per serving

Ingredients

- 800g/1¾lb courgettes/zucchini
- 1 tbsp olive oil
- 300g/11oz raw, shelled king prawns/ jumbo shrimp
- 1 red chilli, deseeded & finely sliced
- 2 onions, sliced
- 2 tbsp freshly chopped coriander/ cilantro
- 2 garlic cloves, crushed
- 1.5l/6 cups chicken stock
- Salt & pepper to taste

Method

1 Top & tail the courgettes and use the shredder blade to turn into thin noodles.

2 Gently heat a large non-stick saucepan on the hob with the olive oil and sauté the prawns, chilli, onions, coriander & garlic for 5-7 minutes until softened.

3 Add the stock & courgette noodles and simmer for 3-5 minutes or until the noodles are tender and the prawns are cooked through.

4 Season and serve.

CHEFS NOTE

Substitute a teaspoon of ground coriander if you don't have fresh coriander to hand.

NO-COOK MELON & CUCUMBER SOUP

165
calories per serving

Ingredients

- 800g/1¾lb cantaloupe melon flesh
- 3 tbsp lime juice
- 3 tbsp olive oil
- Small bunch of fresh mint (thick stalks removed)

- 120ml/½ cup almond milk
- 1 cucumber
- Salt & pepper to taste

Method

1 Place the melon flesh, lime juice, oil, mint & cream in a blender and blend until smooth.

2 Meanwhile top & tail the cucumber and use the shredder blade to turn into thin noodles.

3 Divide the chilled soup into bowls and sit a mound of cucumber noodles on top.

4 Check the seasoning and serve.

CHEFS NOTE

You could also use watermelon to make this soup, but it will have a different texture.

Skinny
SPIRALIZER SOUPS

UNDER 300 CALORIES

PANCETTA & SQUASH NOODLE SOUP

235 calories per serving

Ingredients

- 800g/1¾lb butternut squash
- 100g/3½oz pancetta
- 2 onions, sliced
- 2 garlic cloves, crushed
- 1.5lt/6 cups vegetable or chicken stock
- Low fat cooking oil spray
- Salt & pepper to taste

Method

1 Peel the squash and use the chipper blade to turn into thick spirals.

2 Heat a large non-stick saucepan on the hob with some low fat cooking oil spray and brown the pancetta until it's cooked and crispy. When it's ready, remove from the pan and set to one side.

3 Add the onions and garlic to the saucepan (there should be enough residual oil from the pancetta, if not add a little more) and gently sauté for a few minutes until softened.

4 Add the stock & half of the squash spirals and simmer for 6 minutes.

5 Tip the contents of the pan into a blender and blend until smooth. Return to the pan with the rest of the squash spirals and simmer for another 5-7 minutes or until the squash is tender and the soup is piping hot.

6 Check the seasoning and serve in shallow bowls with the reserved pancetta sprinkled over the top.

CHEFS NOTE

Chop the crispy pancetta finely to make the most of this garnish.

LEEK & POTATO SOUP

255
calories per
serving

Ingredients

- 400g/14oz sweet potatoes
- 1 tbsp olive oil
- 3 leeks, chopped
- 2 garlic cloves, crushed
- 400g/14oz potatoes, peeled & diced
- 1.25lt/5 cups vegetable or chicken stock
- 250ml/1 cup semi skimmed/ half fat milk
- Salt & pepper to taste

Method

1 Peel the sweet potatoes and use the chipper blade to turn into thick spirals.

2 Take a knife and, holding the spirals in bunches, roughly chop into 1cm/½ inch pieces.

3 Heat a large non-stick saucepan on the hob with the olive oil and gently sauté the leeks & garlic for a few minutes until softened.

4 Add the potatoes & stock and cook for 5-7 minutes or until the potatoes are softened.

5 Tip the contents of the saucepan into a blender and pulse until smooth.

6 Return the soup to the pan along with the chopped sweet potato and simmer for 5-7 minutes or until the sweet potato is tender and the soup is piping hot.

7 Stir through the milk, check the seasoning and serve.

CHEFS NOTE

Try serving with some homemade croutons, get the recipe here.

MOROCCAN SOUP

250 calories per serving

Ingredients

- 500g/1lb 2oz butternut squash
- 1 tbsp olive oil
- 1 onion, chopped
- 2 garlic cloves, crushed
- 300g/11oz tinned chickpeas, drained

- 100g/3½oz dried apricots
- 1 tsp ground cinnamon
- 2 tbsp tomato puree
- 1.25lt/5 cups vegetable or chicken stock
- Salt & pepper to taste

Method

1 Peel the squash and use the chipper blade to turn into thick spirals.

2 Take a knife and, holding the spirals in bunches, roughly chop into 1cm/½ inch pieces.

3 Heat a large non-stick saucepan on the hob with the olive oil and gently sauté the onions & garlic for a few minutes until softened.

4 Add the chickpeas, apricots, cinnamon, tomato puree & stock and cook for a few minutes to combine.

5 Tip the contents of the pan into a blender and pulse until smooth.

6 Return to the pan along with the squash and simmer for 5-7 minutes or until the spirals are tender and the soup is piping hot.

7 Combine well. Season and serve.

CHEFS NOTE

This soup benefits from a dash of lemon and some dried chilli flakes to garnish.

JAMBALAYA SOUP

240
calories per
serving

Ingredients

- 800g/1¾lb butternut squash
- 1 tbsp olive oil
- 1 onion, chopped
- 2 garlic cloves, crushed
- 1 green pepper, deseeded & sliced
- 400g/14oz tinned chopped tomatoes
- 2 tbsp Worcestershire sauce
- 1 tsp paprika
- 200g/11oz king prawns/jumbo shrimp
- 1.25lt/5 cups chicken or vegetable stock
- Salt & pepper to taste

Method

1 Peel the squash and use the chipper blade to turn into thick spirals.

2 Take a knife and, holding the spirals in bunches, roughly chop into 1cm/½ inch pieces.

3 Gently heat a large non-stick saucepan on the hob with the olive oil. Add the chopped onions, garlic & peppers and gently sauté for a few minutes until softened.

4 Add the chopped tomatoes, Worcestershire sauce, paprika, prawns, stock & squash and cook for 6-8 minutes or until the prawns are cooked through and the sweet potato is tender.

5 Check the seasoning and serve.

CHEFS NOTE
Try garnishing with a handful of freshly chopped coriander and finely sliced raw red chillies.

KALE & COCONUT MILK CASHEW SOUP

295
calories per
serving

Ingredients

- 600g/1lb 5oz courgettes/zucchini
- 1 tbsp olive oil
- 1 onion, chopped
- 2 garlic cloves, crushed
- 125g/4oz kale, chopped
- 75g/3oz cashew nuts

- 1.25lt/5 cups vegetable or chicken stock
- 200g/7oz frozen peas
- 250ml/1 cup low fat coconut milk
- Salt & pepper to taste

Method

1 Top & tail the courgettes and use the shredder blade to turn into spirals.

2 Heat a large non-stick saucepan on the hob with the olive oil and gently sauté the onions & garlic for a few minutes until softened. Add the kale, nuts & stock and cook for a few minutes.

3 Tip the contents of the saucepan into a blender and pulse until smooth.

4 Return the soup to the pan along with the courgette spirals, peas & coconut milk and simmer for 4-5 minutes or until the spirals are tender and the soup is piping hot.

5 Season and serve.

CHEFS NOTE

The cashew nuts give the soup a creamy texture.

SPICY SQUASH & BROAD BEAN SOUP

270 calories per serving

Ingredients

- 800g/1¾lb butternut squash
- 1 tbsp olive oil
- 1 onion, chopped
- 2 red chillies, deseeded & finely chopped
- 2 garlic cloves, crushed
- ½ tsp ground nutmeg
- 400g/14oz tinned broad beans
- 1.25lt/5 cups chicken or vegetable stock
- Salt & pepper to taste

Method

1 Peel the squash and use the chipper blade to turn into thick spirals.

2 Take a knife and, holding the spirals in bunches, roughly chop into 1cm/½ inch pieces.

3 Gently heat a large non-stick saucepan on the hob with the olive oil. Add the chopped onions, chillies & garlic and gently sauté for a few minutes until softened.

4 Stir through the ground nutmeg. Add the beans, stock & chopped squash and cook for 8-10 minutes or until everything is tender and piping hot.

5 Check the seasoning and serve.

CHEFS NOTE
For a thicker base try blending a couple of ladles of the soup and return to the pan before serving.

BEEF & SHITAKE SPIRAL SOUP

240
calories per serving

Ingredients

- 800g/1¾lb courgettes/zucchini
- 1 tbsp olive oil
- 250g/9oz lean sirloin steak
- 1 onion, sliced
- 4 garlic cloves, crushed
- 200g/7oz shitake mushrooms
- 2 tbsp soy sauce
- 1.5l/6 cups chicken or vegetable stock
- Large bunch spring onions, finely chopped
- Salt & pepper to taste

Method

1 Top & tail the courgettes and use the shredder blade to turn into thin noodles.

2 Heat a large non-stick saucepan on the hob with the olive oil and quickly seal the steak for a minute or two on each side. Remove from the pan and put to one side while you gently sauté the onions, garlic and shitake mushrooms for a few minutes until softened.

3 Once the steak has rested for minute or two, slice finely.

4 Add the soy sauce, stock, steak & noodles and leave to simmer for 4-5 minutes or until the steak is cooked to your liking and the noodles are tender

5 Season and serve with chopped spring onions over the top.

CHEFS NOTE

Adjust the cooking time to suit your own taste (less if you want your steak pink).

TOMATO, LENTIL & CARROT 'RICE' SOUP

215 calories per serving

Ingredients

- 800g/1¾lb carrots
- 1 tbsp olive oil
- 1 onion, sliced
- 2 celery stalks, chopped
- 1 tsp each ground cumin, coriander/cilantro & turmeric
- 2 garlic cloves, crushed
- 400g/14oz tinned chopped tomatoes
- 75g/3oz red lentils
- 1lt/4 cups chicken or vegetable stock
- Salt & pepper to taste

Method

1 Top, tail & peel the carrots and use the shredder blade to turn into thin spirals.

2 Take a knife and, holding the spirals in bunches, roughly chop into 1cm/½ inch pieces.

3 Gently heat a large non-stick saucepan on the hob with the olive oil and sauté the onion, celery & garlic for a few minutes until softened. Add the ground spices, tomatoes, lentil & stock. Stir well, cover and leave to simmer for 20 minutes, stirring occasionally.

4 After this time add the carrot 'rice' and a little more stock to the pan if the soup needs it. Cover and cook for a further 10 minutes or until the lentils are tender.

5 Adjust the seasoning and serve ladled into shallow bowls.

CHEFS NOTE
Adjust the stock in this recipe throughout cooking to get the consistency you prefer.

CARROT 'RICE' & ONION SOUP

225 calories per serving

Ingredients

- 800g/1¾lb carrots
- 1 tbsp olive oil
- 2 onions, sliced
- 2 garlic cloves, crushed
- 2 tsp dried rosemary or oregano
- 400g/7oz potatoes, peeled & diced
- 1.5l/6 cups chicken or vegetable stock
- Salt & pepper to taste

Method

1 Top, tail & peel the carrots and use the shredder blade to turn into thin spirals.

2 Take a knife and, holding the spirals in bunches, roughly chop into 1cm/½ inch pieces.

3 Gently heat a large non-stick saucepan on the hob with the olive oil and sauté the onions, garlic, dried herbs & potatoes for a few minutes until softened. Add the stock and cook for 8 minutes.

4 Tip into a blender and blend for a few seconds until smooth.

5 Return to the pan along with the carrot 'rice' and simmer for 5-7 minutes or until the 'rice' is tender and the soup is piping hot.

6 Season and serve.

CHEFS NOTE

Try adding a handful of tinned beans to the soup before blending to give a thicker base.

CHICKEN & SPRING GREEN SOUP

240 calories per serving

Ingredients

- 800g/1¾lb courgettes/zucchini
- 1 tbsp olive oil
- 1 onion, sliced
- 4 garlic cloves, crushed
- 200g/7oz chicken breast, thinly sliced
- 200g/7oz tinned chickpeas
- 200g/7oz spring greens, shredded
- 1.5l/6 cups chicken or vegetable stock
- 2 tbsp lemon juice
- Salt & pepper to taste

Method

1 Top & tail the courgettes and use the shredder blade to turn into thin noodles.

2 Gently heat a large non-stick saucepan on the hob with the olive oil and sauté the sliced onions & garlic for a few minutes until softened.

3 Add the chicken and cook for 2-3 minutes. Add the chickpeas, greens, stock & noodles and leave to simmer for 5 minutes or until the chicken is cooked through and the soup is piping hot.

4 Divide into bowls and add a dash of lemon juice to each. Season and serve.

CHEFS NOTE
A handful of freshly chopped flat leaf parsley makes a good garnish.

CHICKEN & FRESH CHILLI 'NOODLE' SOUP

210 calories per serving

Ingredients

- 800g/1¾lb courgettes/zucchini
- 1 tbsp olive oil
- 1 onion, sliced
- 2 garlic cloves, crushed
- 1 tsp brown sugar
- 300g/11oz chicken breast, thinly sliced
- 2 red chillies, deeded & sliced
- 1.5lt/6 cups chicken stock
- 3 tbsp freshly chopped coriander/cilantro
- Salt & pepper to taste

Method

1 Top & tail the courgettes and use the shredder blade to turn into thin noodles.

2 Gently heat a large non-stick saucepan on the hob with the olive oil and sauté the sliced onions & garlic for a few minutes until softened.

3 Stir through the sugar and cook for a minute longer before adding the chicken & chillies. Stir-fry for 2-3 minutes, pour in the stock and noodles and leave to simmer for 4-6 minutes or until the chicken is cooked through.

4 Season and serve with the chopped coriander sprinkled over the top.

CHEFS NOTE

Raw red onion and a dash of lime juice make a good garnish to this soup.

PEA & CHICKEN COURGETTE SOUP

265 calories per serving

Ingredients

- 800g/1¾lb courgettes/zucchini
- 1 tbsp olive oil
- 1 onion, finely chopped
- 1 garlic clove, crushed
- ½ red pepper, deseeded & sliced
- 300g/11oz chicken breast, finely sliced
- 300g/11oz frozen peas
- 1.5l/6 cups chicken or vegetable stock
- Salt & pepper to taste

Method

1 Top & tail the courgettes and use the shredder blade to turn into noodles.

2 Gently heat a large non-stick saucepan on the hob with the olive oil. Sauté the onions, garlic & peppers for a few minutes until softened.

3 Add the chicken and cook for 4 minutes. Put the stock, peas & courgettes in the pan and cook 5 minutes or until everything is piping hot.

4 Season and serve.

CHEFS NOTE
Use prawns or pork in place of chicken if you prefer.

CHICKPEA & COURGETTE SOUP

230
calories per serving

Ingredients

- 600g/1lb 5oz courgettes/zucchini
- 1 tbsp olive oil
- 1 onion, chopped
- 2 garlic cloves, crushed
- 500g/1lb 2oz tinned chickpeas, drained
- 1.25lt/5 cups vegetable or chicken stock
- Salt & pepper to taste

Method

1 Top & tail the courgettes and use the shredder blade to turn into spirals.

2 Heat a large non-stick saucepan on the hob with the olive oil and gently sauté the onions & garlic for a few minutes until softened.

3 Tip the sautéed onions, chickpeas and stock into a blender and pulse until smooth.

4 Return to the pan along with the courgette spirals and simmer for 3-5 minutes or until the spirals are tender and the soup is piping hot.

5 Combine well. Season and serve.

CHEFS NOTE

Add more stock to alter the consistency of the soup if you wish.

SWEET POTATO THAI CURRY SOUP

295 calories per serving

Ingredients

- 800g/1¾lb sweet potatoes
- 1 tbsp olive oil
- 1 onion, sliced
- 2 garlic cloves, crushed
- 3 tbsp green Thai curry paste
- 1lt/4 cups chicken or vegetable stock
- 250ml/1 cup low fat coconut milk
- 2 tsp lime juice
- Salt & pepper to taste

Method

1 Peel the sweet potatoes and use the chipper blade to turn into thick spirals.

2 Gently heat a non-stick saucepan on the hob with the olive oil and sauté the onions & garlic for 5 minutes until softened.

3 Stir through the curry paste. Add the stock and sweet potato spirals and simmer for 4-5 minutes.

4 Add the coconut milk and warm through for a couple of minutes until the soup is piping hot and the sweet potato spirals are tender.

5 Stir through the lime juice, season and serve.

CHEFS NOTE
Red Thai curry paste works just as well in this spicy soup.

THAI CHICKEN SOUP

295 calories per serving

Ingredients

- 800g/1¾lb courgettes/zucchini
- 1 tbsp olive oil
- 1 onion, sliced
- 1 garlic clove, crushed
- 2 red peppers, deseeded & sliced
- 200g/7oz chicken breast, thinly sliced
- 3 tbsp Thai red curry paste
- 750ml/3 cups chicken stock
- 250ml/1 cup low fat coconut milk
- 200g/7oz frozen peas
- Lime wedges to serve
- Salt & pepper to taste

Method

1 Top & tail the courgettes and use the shredder blade to turn into thin noodles.

2 Gently heat a large non-stick saucepan on the hob with the olive oil and sauté the sliced onions, garlic & peppers for a few minutes until softened.

3 Add the chicken and cook for 2-3 minutes before stirring through the curry paste.

4 Add the stock, coconut milk, peas & noodles and leave to simmer for 4-5 minutes or until the chicken is cooked through.

5 Season and serve with lime wedges

CHEFS NOTE

It's fine to make this soup with left over chicken. Just shred it up and add to the soup along with the stock.

TURKEY & CARROT SPIRAL SOUP

245 calories per serving

Ingredients

- 800g/1¾lb carrots
- 1 tbsp olive oil
- 300g/11oz turkey breast, thinly sliced
- 2 celery stalks celery, chopped
- 1 onion, sliced
- 2 garlic cloves, crushed
- 3 tbsp freshly chopped basil
- 1.5l/6 cups chicken stock
- Salt & pepper to taste

Method

1 Peel, top & tail the carrots and use the shredder blade to turn into thin spirals.

2 Gently heat a large non-stick saucepan on the hob with the olive oil and sauté the sliced turkey, celery, onion & garlic for 4-5 minutes or until the onions soften.

3 Add the fresh basil, stock & carrot spirals and simmer for 3-5 minutes or until the spirals are tender and the turkey is cooked through.

4 Season and serve.

CHEFS NOTE
Try any fresh chopped herbs you prefer in place of basil.

THICK SWEET POTATO & TOMATO SOUP

260 calories per serving

Ingredients

- 800g/1¾lb sweet potatoes
- 1 tbsp olive oil
- 2 garlic cloves, crushed
- 1 onion, sliced
- 2 tsp turmeric

- 1 tsp each ground cumin & paprika
- ½ tsp salt
- 800g/1¾lb tinned chopped tomatoes
- 500ml/2 cups chicken or vegetable stock
- Salt & pepper to taste

Method

1 Peel the sweet potatoes and use the chipper blade to turn into thick spirals.

2 Gently heat a large non-stick saucepan on the hob with the olive oil and sauté the garlic & onions for a few minutes until softened.

3 Stir through the ground spices, salt, chopped tomatoes, stock & sweet potato spirals.

4 Gently simmer for 5-7 minutes or until the sweet potatoes are tender.

5 Serve and serve.

CHEFS NOTE
Adjust the quantities of tomatoes and stock to get the consistency you prefer.

CHILLI PORK & GREEN BEAN SOUP

230 calories per serving

Ingredients

- 600g/1lb 5oz courgettes/zucchini
- 1 tbsp olive oil
- 300g/11oz pork tenderloin, sliced into strips
- 1-2 red chillies, deseeded & finely chopped
- 2 garlic cloves, crushed
- 1 onion, sliced
- 200g/7oz green beans, chopped
- 1.5l/6 cups chicken or vegetable stock
- Salt & pepper to taste

Method

1 Top & tail the courgettes and use the shredder blade to turn into thin noodles.

2 Gently heat a large non-stick large saucepan on the hob with the olive oil and sauté the pork, garlic, chopped chillies, onions & green beans for 3-5 minutes until softened.

3 Add the stock and courgette noodles and simmer for 3-5 minutes or until the noodles are tender and the pork is cooked through.

4 Serve in a shallow bowl with the spring onions over the top.

CHEFS NOTE
Use one or two red chillies depending on your preference.

CHICKEN & COCONUT MILK 'NOODLE' SOUP

265 calories per serving

Ingredients

- 800g/1¾lb courgettes/zucchini
- 1 tbsp olive oil
- 1 onion, sliced
- 1 garlic clove, crushed
- 1 tsp each ground ginger & coriander/cilantro

- 300g/11oz chicken breast, thinly sliced
- 500ml/2 cups chicken stock
- 500ml/2 cups low fat coconut milk
- 2 tbsp fish sauce
- Lime wedges to serve
- Salt & pepper to taste

Method

1 Top & tail the courgettes and use the shredder blade to turn into thin noodles.

2 Gently heat a large non-stick saucepan on the hob with the olive oil and sauté the sliced onions & garlic for a few minutes until softened.

3 Stir through the ginger & coriander and cook for a minute longer before adding the chicken. Cook for 2-3 minutes, pour in the stock, noodles, coconut milk & fish sauce and leave to simmer for 4-5 minutes or until the chicken is cooked through.

4 Season and serve with lime wedges.

CHEFS NOTE

Finely slice some green chillies as a garnish to give this soup a fiery finish.

HAM & CARROT SOUP

270
calories per
serving

Ingredients

- 800g/1¾lb carrots
- 1 tbsp olive oil
- 1 onion, sliced
- 1 garlic clove, crushed
- 2 tsp dried basil

- 400g/7oz potatoes, peeled & diced
- 1.5l/6 cups chicken or vegetable stock
- 200g/7oz cooked ham, shredded
- Salt & pepper to taste

Method

1 Top, tail & peel the carrots and use the shredder blade to turn into thin spirals.

2 Take a knife and, holding the spirals in bunches, roughly chop into 1cm/½ inch pieces.

3 Gently heat a large non-stick saucepan on the hob with the olive oil and sauté the onion, garlic, basil & potatoes for a few minutes until softened.

4 Add the stock and cook for 6-8 minutes or until the potatoes are tender.

5 Tip the contents of the pan into a blender and blend until smooth.

6 Return to the pan along with the carrot 'rice' & shredded ham and simmer for 5-7 minutes or until the 'rice' is tender and the soup is piping hot.

7 Season and serve.

CHEFS NOTE
This is also good with sweet potato or squash 'rice' in place of the carrots.

Skinny
SPIRALIZER SOUPS

UNDER 400 CALORIES

HADDOCK & HORSERADISH SOUP

390
calories per serving

Ingredients

- 400g/14oz sweet potatoes
- 2 carrots, chopped
- 1.25lt/5 cups semi skimmed/half fat milk
- 2 tbsp horseradish sauce
- 400g/14oz white potatoes, peeled & diced
- 250g/9oz smoked haddock, cubed
- 3 tbsp freshly chopped flat leaf parsley
- Salt & pepper to taste

Method

1 Peel the sweet potatoes and use the chipper blade to turn into thick spirals.

2 Take a knife and, holding the spirals in bunches, roughly chop into 1cm/½ inch pieces.

3 Heat a large non-stick saucepan with the carrots, milk, horseradish & white potatoes and gently cook for a few minutes until the potatoes are softened.

4 Tip the contents of the saucepan into a blender and pulse until smooth.

5 Return the soup to the pan along with the chopped sweet potato & haddock. Gently simmer for 5-7 minutes or until the sweet potato is tender & the fish is cooked through.

6 Sprinkle with chopped parsley and serve.

CHEFS NOTE
Use boneless haddock fillets for this soup.

SPLIT PEA, BACON & POTATO 'RICE' SOUP

395 calories per serving

Ingredients

- 800g/1¾lb potatoes
- 200g/7oz lean, back bacon
- 1 onion, sliced
- 2 carrots, chopped
- 2 celery stalks, chopped
- 2 garlic cloves, crushed
- 125g/4oz red lentils
- 1.5lt/6 cups vegetable or chicken stock
- Low fat cooking oil spray
- Salt & pepper to taste

Method

1 Peel the potatoes and use the shredder blade to turn into thin spirals.

2 Take a knife and, holding the spirals in bunches, roughly chop into 1cm/½ inch pieces.

3 Heat a large non-stick saucepan on the hob with some low fat cooking oil spray and cook the bacon until it's brown and crispy. When it's ready, remove from the pan, set to one side and finely chop.

4 Add the onions, carrots, celery and garlic to the saucepan (there should be enough residual oil from the bacon, if not add a little more) and gently sauté for a few minutes until softened.

5 Add the lentils & stock. Combine well, cover and leave to simmer for 20 minutes, stirring occasionally.

6 After this time add a little more stock to the pan if the soup needs it. Add the potatoes, cover and cook for a further 10 minutes or until the lentils and potatoes are all tender.

7 Adjust the seasoning and serve ladled into shallow bowls with the chopped bacon over the top

CHEFS NOTE
Add more stock if you need to loosen the soup up a little.

AROMATIC CHICKEN 'RICE' SOUP

365 calories per serving

Ingredients

- 400g/14oz sweet potatoes
- 1 tbsp olive oil
- 1 leek, finely chopped
- 2 celery stalks, chopped
- 2 carrots, finely chopped
- 1 tsp each ground cumin, coriander & turmeric
- 4 tbsp raisins, chopped
- 2 tbsp honey
- 250g/9oz cooked chicken breast, finely shredded
- 1.5lt/6 cups vegetable or chicken stock
- 4 tbsp fat free Greek yogurt
- Salt & pepper to taste

Method

1 Peel the sweet potatoes and use the chipper blade to turn into thick spirals.

2 Take a knife and, holding the spirals in bunches, roughly chop into 1cm/½ inch pieces.

3 Heat a large non-stick saucepan on the hob with the olive oil and gently sauté the leek, celery & carrots for a few minutes until softened.

4 Stir through the ground spices and add the raisins, honey, chicken, stock & chopped sweet potato. Simmer for 6-8 minutes or until the sweet potato is tender and the soup is piping hot.

5 Check the seasoning and serve with a dollop of yogurt in the centre.

CHEFS NOTE

You could add half a teaspoon of chilli powder to this warming soup if you wish.

SALMON & COCONUT MILK SOUP

320 calories per serving

Ingredients

- 800g/1¾lb courgettes/zucchini
- 1 tbsp olive oil
- 300g/11oz skinless, boneless salmon fillet
- 1 onion, sliced
- 1 garlic clove, crushed
- 2 tbsp tomato puree
- 500ml/2 cups chicken stock
- 500ml/2 cups low fat coconut milk
- 2 tbsp freshly chopped coriander/cilantro
- Salt & pepper to taste

Method

1 Top & tail the courgettes and use the shredder blade to turn into thin noodles.

2 Gently heat a large non-stick saucepan on the hob with the olive oil and quickly fry the salmon for 2 minutes on each side to seal.

3 Add the sliced onions & garlic and sauté for a few minutes until softened. After this time gently break the fish apart into flakes using a fork.

4 Stir through the puree, stock, noodles & coconut milk and leave to simmer for 4-5 minutes or until the salmon is cooked through and the noodles are tender

5 Season and serve with chopped coriander over the top.

CHEFS NOTE
Avoid stirring the soup too much when cooking as you don't want the salmon flakes to break apart completely.

SPANISH SWEET POTATO SOUP

320
calories per serving

Ingredients

- 800g/1¾lb sweet potatoes
- 1 red onion, chopped
- 1 tbsp olive oil
- 2 garlic cloves, crushed
- 125g/4oz sliced chorizo sausage, chopped

- 2 tbsp tomato puree/paste
- 1 tsp paprika
- 1lt/4 cups chicken or vegetable stock
- 200g/7oz tinned chopped tomatoes
- Salt & pepper to taste

Method

1 Peel the sweet potatoes and use the chipper blade to turn into thick spirals.

2 Gently heat a large non-stick saucepan on the hob with the olive oil. Add the chopped red onions, garlic & chorizo and gently sauté for a few minutes until softened.

3 Stir through the puree and paprika. Add the stock & chopped tomatoes and cook for 2 minutes.

4 Add the spirals and cook for 5-7 minutes or until the spirals are tender and the soup is piping hot.

5 Check the seasoning and serve.

CHEFS NOTE

Add some more paprika and a little chopped flat leaf parsley to garnish.

SWEET POTATO & KIDNEY BEAN SOUP

350 calories per serving

Ingredients

- 600g/1lb 5oz sweet potatoes
- 1 tbsp olive oil
- 1 onion, chopped
- 2 garlic cloves, crushed
- 1 red pepper, sliced
- 2 tbsp tomato puree/paste
- 2 tsp dried oregano
- 300g/11oz tinned kidney beans
- 1.25lt/5 cups chicken or vegetable stock
- 200g/7oz tinned chopped tomatoes
- ½ avocado, peeled & diced
- 1 tbsp lime juice
- Salt & pepper to taste

Method

1 Peel the sweet potatoes and use the chipper blade to turn into thick spirals.

2 Take a knife and, holding the spirals in bunches, roughly chop into 1cm/½ inch pieces.

3 Gently heat a large non-stick saucepan on the hob with the olive oil. Add the chopped onions, garlic & peppers and gently sauté for a few minutes until softened.

4 Stir through the puree and oregano. Add the kidney beans, stock, chopped tomatoes and sweet potatoes and cook for 8-10 minutes or until everything is tender and piping hot.

5 Mix the avocado with the lime juice and serve the soup in shallow bowls with the lime avocado cubes piled into the centre of each.

CHEFS NOTE
Shredded chicken makes a good addition to this hearty soup.

SHREDDED CHICKEN & SWEET POTATO 'RICE' SOUP

320 calories per serving

Ingredients

- 800g/1¾lb sweet potatoes
- 1 tbsp olive oil
- 1 onion, chopped
- 2 celery stalks, chopped
- 2 garlic cloves, crushed

- 1 tsp dried thyme
- 1 tsp freshly grated ginger
- 1.25lt/5 cups chicken or vegetable stock
- 250g/9oz cooked shredded chicken
- Salt & pepper to taste

Method

1 Peel the sweet potatoes and use the chipper blade to turn into thick spirals.

2 Take a knife and, holding the spirals in bunches, roughly chop into 1cm/½ inch pieces.

3 Gently heat a large non-stick saucepan on the hob with the olive oil. Add the chopped onions, celery, garlic, thyme & ginger and gently sauté for a few minutes until softened.

4 Add the stock and sweet potatoes and cook for 5 minutes. Add the shredded chicken and cook for 3-5 minutes longer or until the sweet potato is tender and the chicken is piping hot.

5 Check the seasoning and serve.

CHEFS NOTE
Try rosemary or mixed dried herbs instead of thyme.

Skinny
SPIRALIZER SOUP

STOCK

It's not necessary to make your own stock to create good soup, quality shop-bought stock works well too. However if you do want to have a go at making homemade stock here are some basic recipes.

BASIC VEGETABLE STOCK

Ingredients

- 1 tbsp olive oil
- 1 onion, chopped
- 1 leek, chopped
- 1 carrot, chopped
- 1 small bulb fennel, chopped
- 3 garlic cloves, crushed
- 1 tbsp black peppercorns

- 75g/3oz mushrooms
- 2 sticks celery, chopped
- 3 tomatoes, diced
- 2 tbsp freshly chopped flat leaf parsley
- 2 bay leaves
- 3lt/12 cups water

Method

1 Gently sauté the onions, leeks, carrots and fennel in the olive oil for a few minutes in a large lidded saucepan.

2 Add all the other ingredients, cover and bring to the boil. Leave to gently simmer for 20 minutes with the lid on.

3 Cool for a little while. Pour the contents through a sieve and store the finished stock liquid in the fridge for a couple of days or freeze in batches.

BASIC CHICKEN STOCK

Ingredients

- 1 tbsp olive oil
- 1 left over roast chicken carcass
- 2 carrots, chopped
- 2 onions, halved
- 2 stalks celery, chopped

- 10 black peppercorns
- 2 bay leaves
- 2 tbsp freshly chopped parsley
- 1 tsp freshly chopped thyme
- 3lt/12 cups water

Method

1 Gently sauté the onions, carrots and celery in the olive oil for a few minutes in a large lidded saucepan.

2 Break the chicken carcass up into pieces and add to the pan along with all the other ingredients, cover and bring to the boil. Leave to very gently simmer for 1hr with the lid on.

3 Cool for a little while. Pour the contents through a sieve and store the finished stock liquid in the fridge for a couple of days or freeze in batches. You may find you need to skim a little fat from the top of the stock after cooking.

BASIC FISH STOCK

Ingredients

- 1 tbsp olive oil
- 450g/1lb fish bones, heads carcasses etc (avoid oily fish when making stock)
- 4 leeks, chopped
- 1 fennel bulb, chopped
- 4 carrots, chopped
- 2 tbsp freshly chopped parsley
- 250ml/1 cup dry white wine
- 2.5lt/10 cups water

Method

1 Gently sauté the carrots, leeks and fennel in the olive oil for a few minutes in a large lidded saucepan.

2 Clean the fish bones to ensure there is no blood as this can 'spoil' the stock. Add all the other ingredients, cover and bring to the boil. Leave to very gently simmer for 1hr with the lid on.

3 Cool for a little while. Pour the contents through a sieve and store the finished stock liquid in the fridge for a couple of days or freeze in batches. You may find you need to skim a little fat from the top of the stock after cooking.

Skinny
SPIRALIZER
SOUP

GARNISH IDEAS & EXTRAS

These are some lovely garnish ideas which will complement your soups. You'll need to use your spiralizer for some of these, but not all.

SPICED SWEDE SPRINKLES

30
calories per portion

Ingredients

- 400g/14oz swede/turnip
- 1 tbsp olive oil
- 1 tsp crushed sea salt flakes
- 2 tsp chilli powder

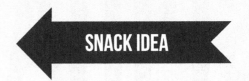

SNACK IDEA

Method

1 Preheat the oven to 350f/180c/Gas 4

2 Peel the swede and use the straight/slicer blade to turn into thick ribbons/slices. Dry off the ribbons really well using kitchen towels.

3 Combine everything together and spread out onto a greaseproof baking tray.

4 Place into the oven and cook for 15-25 minutes or until the swede pieces turn golden & crisp (keep an eye on the temperature, you don't want the edges burning before the inner part is cooked)

5 Allow to cool and finely chop.

CHEFS NOTE

This is lovely as a garnish but also good as a snack if you leave the chips un-chopped.

HOMEMADE CROUTONS

50
calories per portion

Ingredients

- 4 slices thick wholemeal bread
- 2 tsp garlic powder
- 2 tsp dried mixed herbs
- 1 tsp crushed sea salt flakes
- Low cal cooking oil spray

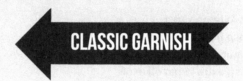

CLASSIC GARNISH

Method

1 Preheat the oven to 350f/180c/Gas 4

2 Remove the crusts with a knife and cube the bread into crouton-sized pieces.

3 Spray the bread cubes with some low cal oil and place in a plastic bag with the garlic powder, herbs and salt. Give the bag a good shake until all the bread is covered with the seasoning.

4 Lay the bread cubes out on a non-stick baking tray and cook in the preheated oven for 13-15 minutes or until the croutons are crisp and golden brown.

CHEFS NOTE
You could add some grated Parmesan to the seasoning for extra taste.

EASY GREMOLATA

22
calories per
portion

Ingredients

- 4 tbsp lemon zest
- 3 tbsp freshly chopped flat leaf parsley
- 4 garlic cloves, crushed
- 1 tbsp extra virgin olive oil
- ½ tsp crushed seas salt flakes

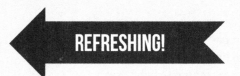
REFRESHING!

Method

1 Mix everything together until really well combined.
Try using a small clean lidded jar and shaking.

2 Add a little more oil if needed and feel free to alter
the balance of salt, garlic and lemon to suit your
own taste.

CHEFS NOTE

This is great sprinkled or stirred through
soup just prior serving.

BALSAMIC ONIONS

35
calories per
portion

Ingredients

- 1 tbsp olive oil
- 2 red onions, sliced
- 1 tsp brown sugar
- 1 tbsp balsamic vinegar

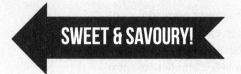

SWEET & SAVOURY!

Method

1 Heat the olive oil in a non-stick frying pan and gently sauté for 10-15 minutes until softened and browned.

2 Stir through the brown sugar and vinegar. Increase the heat and cook for 2 minutes longer.

3 Remove from the pan and store in the fridge for up to three days.

CHEFS NOTE

Stirred through soup just before serving, this garnish adds a lovely sweet taste.

SPICED PUMPKIN SEEDS

70
calories per portion

Ingredients

- 100g/3½oz pumpkin seeds
- 1 tbsp olive oil
- ½ tsp each garlic powder, salt, ground cumin & coriander/cilantro

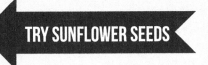

TRY SUNFLOWER SEEDS

Method

1 Preheat the oven to 350f/180c/Gas 4

2 Combine everything together and spread onto a greaseproof baking tray.

3 Place into the oven and cook for 8-12 minutes or until golden, crisp and cooked through.

4 Allow to cool and store in an airtight container for up to a week.

CHEFS NOTE

These can be sprinkled whole or chopped before adding as a garnish. A teaspoon of brown sugar makes a good addition to the seeds too.

BAKED SWEET POTATO CHIPS

55 calories per portion

Ingredients

- 400g/14oz sweet potatoes
- 1 tbsp olive oil
- 1 tsp crushed sea salt flakes
- ½ tsp each paprika, cumin & chilli powder

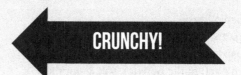

CRUNCHY!

Method

1 Preheat the oven to 350f/180c/Gas 4

2 Peel the sweet potatoes and use the straight/ slicer blade to turn into thick ribbons/slices. Dry off the ribbons really well using kitchen towels.

3 Combine everything together and spread out onto a greaseproof baking tray.

4 Place into the oven and cook for 10-15 minutes or until the sweet potato turns golden & crisp (keep an eye on the temperature, you don't want the edges burning before the inner part is cooked)

5 Allow to cool and finely chop.

CHEFS NOTE
Sprinkle over soup to serve as a crunchy garnish.

SPICED POPPED CORN GARNISH

45 calories per portion

Ingredients

- 1 tbsp olive oil
- 50g/2oz popping corn
- 1 tbsp low fat 'butter' spread
- 1 tsp each garlic powder, salt & paprika

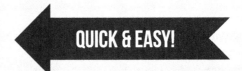

QUICK & EASY!

Method

1 Heat the olive oil in a non-stick lidded saucepan.

2 When the oil is good and hot, add the corn and continue to heat until the corn stops popping.

3 Combine with the rest of the ingredients and serve as an unusual and tasty soup garnish.

CHEFS NOTE
If you want the corn broken up a little, place in a bag and bash a few times with a rolling pin.

GROUND SPICE YOGURT

40
calories per portion

Ingredients

- 5 tbsp fat free Greek yogurt
- 1 tsp turmeric
- 1 tsp paprika
- ½ tsp cumin
- ½ tsp ground coriander/cilantro

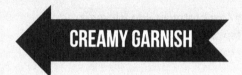
CREAMY GARNISH

Method

1 Combine all the ingredients together and store in the fridge until ready to use.

2 Dollop a spoonful in the centre of any smooth soup you like and gently stir through.

CHEFS NOTE
Feel free to alter the balance of spices in this simple garnish and try some freshly chopped herbs too if you like.

SALTY ROASTED SQUASH SEEDS

20
calories per portion

Ingredients

- 125g/4oz butternut squash seeds
- 1-2 tsp crushed sea salt flakes
- Low cal cooking oil spray

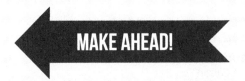

MAKE AHEAD!

Method

1 Preheat the oven to 350f/180c/Gas 4

2 Cover the seeds with a little low cal spray and spread out on a baking tray.

3 Place into the oven and cook for 8-12 minutes or until crisp.

4 Sprinkle with salt while they are still hot. Combine well and allow to cool.

5 Use straight away or store in an airtight container for up to a week.

CHEFS NOTE

This is a great way of using up the left over seeds from any squash spiralizing recipe. Young, tender seeds give the best result.

TOASTED PINE NUTS & PARSLEY

90
calories per portion

Ingredients

- 4 tbsp pine nuts
- 3 tbsp freshly chopped flat leaf parsley
- ½ tsp crushed sea salt flakes

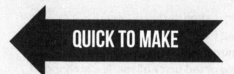

QUICK TO MAKE

Method

1 Gently heat a non-stick frying pan on the hob. Add the pine nuts and cook for 2-4 minutes or until the colour begins to change.

2 Move around the pan frequently and don't allow the nuts to burn.

3 When cooked toss with the salt and finely chopped parsley.

4 Serve sprinkled over soup.

CHEFS NOTE

This works best with a smooth based soup. Chop the nuts if you want a finer garnish.

OLIVE & CORIANDER GREMOLATA

40
calories per portion

Ingredients

- 2 tbsp lemon zest
- 3 tbsp freshly chopped coriander/ cilantro
- 3 tbsp pitted black olives, finely chopped
- 4 garlic cloves, crushed
- 1 tbsp extra virgin olive oil
- ½ tsp crushed seas salt flakes

Method

1 Mix everything together until really well combined. Try using a small clean lidded jar and shaking.

2 Add a little more oil if needed and feel free to alter the balance of salt, garlic and lemon to suit your own taste.

CHEFS NOTE

This is quite a robust garnish, use it with subtly flavoured or Asian inspired soups.

BONUS

SPIRALIZER MEAL RECIPES

If you want to get even more out of your spiralizer try 'The Skinny Spiralizer Recipe Book' also by CookNation.

This bonus section contains eight recipes taken from that best selling title.

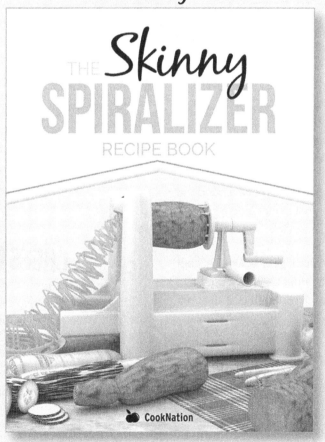

CREAMY THAI VEG NOODLES

320 calories per serving

Ingredients

- 1 courgette/zucchini weighing 150g/5oz
- 1 carrot weighing 150g/5oz
- 1 garlic clove, crushed
- 1 tsp grated ginger
- 1 tsp lemon juice
- 1 tbsp soy sauce
- ½ ripe avocado
- 60ml/¼ cup water
- Low cal cooking oil spray
- Salt & pepper to taste

Method

1 Top & tail the courgette. Peel the carrot and use the shredder blade to turn both into thin noodles.

2 Gently heat a large non-stick frying pan on the hob with a little low cal oil.

3 Add the courgette noodles and move around the pan for 3-5 minutes or until tender (add a splash of water to the pan if you need to).

4 Meanwhile place all the other ingredients, except the carrot, into a mini blender to make a creamy dressing (or mash everything together with a fork if you don't have one).

5 Take the pan off the heat. Stir through the creamy dressing and toss the carrot through.

6 Season and serve.

CHEFS NOTE

The raw carrots give this dish a nice crunch, it's fine to sauté though if you prefer.

GRILLED COD ON A BED OF SPIRALS

270 calories per serving

Ingredients

- 1 courgette/zucchini weighing 200g/11oz
- 1 carrot weighing 200g/11oz
- 150g/5oz skinless, boneless cod loin
- Zest & juice of ¼ lemon
- 1 tbsp low fat 'butter' spread
- Low cal cooking oil spray
- Salt & pepper to taste

Method

1 Preheat the grill to a medium/high heat.

2 Top & tail the courgette, peel the carrot and use the shredder blade to turn into thin spirals.

3 Season the cod, spray with a little low cal oil and brush with the zest and lemon juice.

4 Place under the preheated grill and, turning once, cook for 8-10 minutes or until the fish is cooked through.

5 Meanwhile gently heat the 'butter' in a non-stick frying pan. Add the courgette and carrot spirals and cook for 3-4 minutes or until tender.

6 Arrange the cooked vegetables on a plate, sit the grilled cod on top. Season and serve.

CHEFS NOTE
Serve with lemon wedges.

SHRIMP & FRESH PEA NOODLES

260 calories per serving

Ingredients

- Courgettes/zucchini weighing 300g/11oz
- ½ onion, sliced
- ½ red pepper, deseeded & sliced
- 1 garlic clove, crushed
- A pinch of crushed dried chillies
- 150g/5oz raw, shelled king prawns/ jumbo shrimp
- 1 tbsp soy sauce
- 2 tsp Thai fish sauce
- 1 tsp lime juice
- 75g/3oz fresh peas
- Low cal cooking oil spray
- Salt & pepper to taste

Method

1 Top & tail the courgettes and use the shredder blade to turn into spaghetti noodles.

2 Gently heat a large non-stick frying pan on the hob with a little low cal oil. Sauté the onion, peppers & garlic for a few minutes until softened.

3 Add the chillies, prawns, soy sauce, fish sauce & lime juice and cook for 3 minutes.

4 Add the noodles & fresh peas and move around the pan for 3-5 minutes or until everything is piping hot.

5 Season and serve.

CHEFS NOTE

Use chicken instead of prawns if you prefer.

SWEET ROASTED CHERRY TOMATO & ZUCCHINI SPIRALS

270 calories per serving

Ingredients

- Courgettes/zucchini weighing 300g/11oz
- 200g/7oz ripe cherry tomatoes
- 1 tsp brown sugar (or honey)
- 2 garlic cloves, crushed
- ½ onion, chopped
- 1 tbsp olive oil
- 1 tbsp freshly chopped basil
- Low cal cooking oil spray
- Salt & pepper to taste

Method

1 Preheat the oven to 200c/400f/Gas 6.

2 Halve the cherry tomatoes, place on a baking tray, spray with a little low cal oil and sprinkle with sugar. Put into the oven and cook for about 20 minutes or until they are roasted and soft.

3 Meanwhile top & tail the courgettes and use the chipper blade to turn into thick spirals.

4 Gently heat a large non-stick frying pan on the hob with the garlic, onion & olive oil and sauté for a few minutes until softened.

5 Add the spirals and move around the pan for 3-5 minutes or until everything is piping hot. Toss through the sweet roasted tomatoes and pile into a shallow bowl.

6 Sprinkle with basil. Season and serve.

CHEFS NOTE
Vine ripened plum tomatoes will work just as well but you may need to roast for a little longer.

BEEF KEEMA

360
calories per
serving

Ingredients

- 1 courgette/zucchini weighing 200g/11oz
- 1 carrot weighing 200g/11oz
- 1 tsp olive oil
- ½ onion, sliced
- 1 garlic clove, crushed
- 125g/4oz lean mince/ground beef
- ½ tsp garam masala
- 1 tsp turmeric
- Large pinch of sea salt
- 100g/3½oz tinned chopped tomatoes
- Low cal cooking oil spray
- Salt & pepper to taste

Method

1 Peel the carrot. Top & tail the courgette & carrot and use the shredder blade to turn both into thin spirals.

2 Heat a non-stick frying pan with the olive oil and sauté the onion & garlic for a few minutes. Add the beef and brown for a couple of minutes.

3 Stir through the garam masala, turmeric & salt and cook for 2 minutes. Add the tomatoes and spirals.

4 Cover and leave to simmer for 5 minutes or until the beef is cooked through and the spirals are tender. Season and serve.

CHEFS NOTE

Chopped coriander and chillies make a good garnish for this simple Indian dish.

CHICKEN & COURGETTE SKEWERS

360 calories per serving

Ingredients

- Courgettes/zucchini weighing 300g/11oz
- 1 tbsp olive oil
- ½ red chilli, deseeded & finely chopped
- Zest & juice of ½ lime
- Large pinch of sea salt
- 125g/4oz chicken breast, cubed
- 1 tsp honey
- Low cal cooking oil spray
- Metal kebab skewers
- Salt & pepper to taste

Method

1 Preheat the grill to a medium/high heat.

2 Top & Tail the courgettes and use the slicer/ straight blade to turn into ribbons.

3 Place the ribbons in a bowl with the olive oil, chilli, lime juice, zest, and salt. Combine really well to coat every inch of the courgette in the olive oil.

4 Meanwhile season the chicken and, in a bowl, combine with the honey.

5 Place the chicken cubes and courgette in turn on the skewers to make 1 large or two smaller kebabs.

6 Place under the preheated grill and, turning occasionally, cook for 8-10 minutes or until the chicken is cooked through.

CHEFS NOTE
Skewer the ribbons by weaving them concertina style on the kebab sticks.

FRESH TUNA STIR-FRY

360
calories per
serving

Ingredients

- Carrots weighing 300g/11oz
- 75g/3oz asparagus spears
- 150g/5oz fresh tuna steak
- 1 tbsp soy sauce
- 1 tsp honey
- 1 tsp lime juice
- 2 radishes, sliced
- 1 handful watercress
- Salt & pepper to taste

Method

1 Top, tail & peel the carrots and use the straight/slicer blade to turn into thin ribbons.

2 Gently heat a large non-stick frying pan on the hob with the olive oil and sauté the carrot and asparagus for 2 minutes.

3 Make some room in the pan, add the tuna steak and cook for 1 minute each side (pile the veg on top of the tuna steak if you find it's cooking too fast)

4 Meanwhile mix together the soy sauce, honey & lime juice and pour this over the tuna and veg.

5 Tip everything onto a plate with the watercress on the side. Season and serve.

CHEFS NOTE

Increase the cooking time for the tuna if you don't want rare steak.

CHUNKY CHICKPEA 'PASTA'

310 calories per serving

Ingredients

- Courgettes/zucchini weighing 300g/11oz
- ½ onion, chopped
- 1 garlic clove, crushed
- 200g/7oz tinned chickpeas, drained
- 250ml/1 cup vegetable stock
- Low cal cooking oil spray
- Salt & pepper to taste

Method

1 Top & tail the courgettes and use the shredder blade to turn into spaghetti noodles.

2 Heat a large non-stick frying pan on the hob with a little low cal spray and gently sauté the onions & garlic for a few minutes until softened.

3 Meanwhile gently warm the chickpeas in a small pan with the stock.

4 Tip the sautéed onions into a blender and use a slotted spoon to add the chickpeas too. Add about half the stock and pulse for a second at a time until you have a chunky sauce. Add more of the stock to alter the consistency if you want.

5 Add the spaghetti noodles to the empty frying pan and move around the pan for 3-5 minutes or until they are piping hot. Tip over the chickpea sauce.

6 Combine well. Season and serve.

CHEFS NOTE
Garnish with chopped flat leaf parsley.

CONVERSION CHART: DRY INGREDIENTS

Metric	Imperial
7g	¼ oz
15g	½ oz
20g	¾ oz
25g	1 oz
40g	1½oz
50g	2oz
60g	2½oz
75g	3oz
100g	3½oz
125g	4oz
140g	4½oz
150g	5oz
165g	5½oz
175g	6oz
200g	7oz
225g	8oz
250g	9oz
275g	10oz
300g	11oz
350g	12oz
375g	13oz
400g	14oz

Metric	Imperial
425g	15oz
450g	1lb
500g	1lb 2oz
550g	1¼lb
600g	1lb 5oz
650g	1lb 7oz
675g	1½lb
700g	1lb 9oz
750g	1lb 11oz
800g	1¾lb
900g	2lb
1kg	2¼lb
1.1kg	2½lb
1.25kg	2¾lb
1.35kg	3lb
1.5kg	3lb 6oz
1.8kg	4lb
2kg	4½lb
2.25kg	5lb
2.5kg	5½lb
2.75kg	6lb

CONVERSION CHART: LIQUID MEASURES

Metric	Imperial	US
25ml	1fl oz	
60ml	2fl oz	¼ cup
75ml	2½ fl oz	
100ml	3½fl oz	
120ml	4fl oz	½ cup
150ml	5fl oz	
175ml	6fl oz	
200ml	7fl oz	
250ml	8½ fl oz	1 cup
300ml	10½ fl oz	
360ml	12½ fl oz	
400ml	14fl oz	
450ml	15½ fl oz	
600ml	1 pint	
750ml	1¼ pint	3 cups
1 litre	1½ pints	4 cups

Other
COOKNATION
TITLES

If you enjoyed 'The Skinny Spiralizer Soup Recipe Book' we'd really appreciate your feedback. Reviews help others decide if this is the right book for them so a moment of your time would be appreciated.

Thank you.

You may also be interested in other '**Skinny**' titles in the CookNation series. You can find all the following great titles by searching under '**CookNation**'.

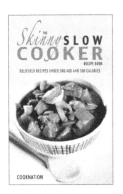

THE SKINNY SLOW COOKER RECIPE BOOK

Delicious Recipes Under 300, 400 And 500 Calories.

Paperback / eBook

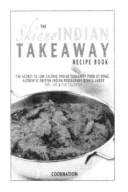

THE SKINNY INDIAN TAKEAWAY RECIPE BOOK

Authentic British Indian Restaurant Dishes Under 300, 400 And 500 Calories. The Secret To Low Calorie Indian Takeaway Food At Home.

Paperback / eBook

THE HEALTHY KIDS SMOOTHIE BOOK

40 Delicious Goodness In A Glass Recipes for Happy Kids.

eBook

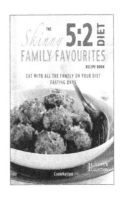

THE SKINNY 5:2 FAST DIET FAMILY FAVOURITES RECIPE BOOK

Eat With All The Family On Your Diet Fasting Days.

Paperback / eBook

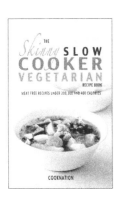

THE SKINNY SLOW COOKER VEGETARIAN RECIPE BOOK

40 Delicious Recipes Under 200, 300 And 400 Calories.

Paperback / eBook

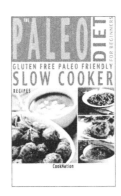

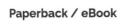

THE PALEO DIET FOR BEGINNERS SLOW COOKER RECIPE BOOK

Gluten Free, Everyday Essential Slow Cooker Paleo Recipes For Beginners.

eBook

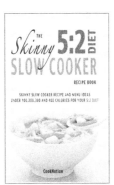

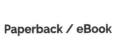

THE SKINNY 5:2 SLOW COOKER RECIPE BOOK

Skinny Slow Cooker Recipe And Menu Ideas Under 100, 200, 300 & 400 Calories For Your 5:2 Diet.

Paperback / eBook

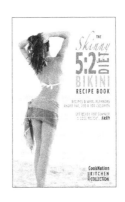

THE SKINNY 5:2 BIKINI DIET RECIPE BOOK

Recipes & Meal Planners Under 100, 200 & 300 Calories. Get Ready For Summer & Lose Weight...FAST!

Paperback / eBook

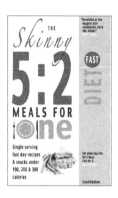

THE SKINNY 5:2 FAST DIET MEALS FOR ONE

Single Serving Fast Day Recipes & Snacks Under 100, 200 & 300 Calories.

Paperback / eBook

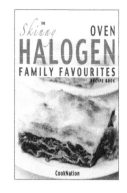

THE SKINNY HALOGEN OVEN FAMILY FAVOURITES RECIPE BOOK

Healthy, Low Calorie Family Meal-Time Halogen Oven Recipes Under 300, 400 and 500 Calories.

Paperback / eBook

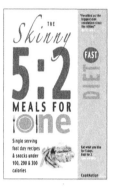

THE SKINNY 5:2 FAST DIET VEGETARIAN MEALS FOR ONE

Single Serving Fast Day Recipes & Snacks Under 100, 200 & 300 Calories.

Paperback / eBook

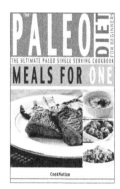

THE PALEO DIET FOR BEGINNERS MEALS FOR ONE

The Ultimate Paleo Single Serving Cookbook.

Paperback / eBook

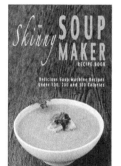

THE SKINNY SOUP MAKER RECIPE BOOK

Delicious Low Calorie, Healthy and Simple Soup Recipes Under 100, 200 and 300 Calories. Perfect For Any Diet and Weight Loss Plan.

Paperback / eBook

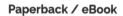

THE PALEO DIET FOR BEGINNERS HOLIDAYS

Thanksgiving, Christmas & New Year Paleo Friendly Recipes.
eBook

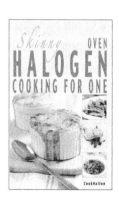

SKINNY HALOGEN OVEN COOKING FOR ONE

Single Serving, Healthy, Low Calorie Halogen Oven RecipesUnder 200, 300 and 400 Calories.

Paperback / eBook

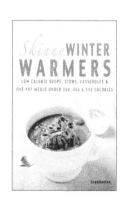

SKINNY WINTER WARMERS RECIPE BOOK

Soups, Stews, Casseroles & One Pot Meals Under 300, 400 & 500 Calories.

Paperback / eBook

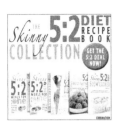

THE SKINNY 5:2 DIET RECIPE BOOK COLLECTION

All The 5:2 Fast Diet Recipes You'll Ever Need. All Under 100, 200, 300, 400 And 500 Calories.

eBook

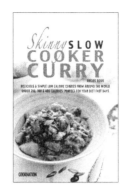

THE SKINNY SLOW COOKER CURRY RECIPE BOOK

Low Calorie Curries From Around The World.

Paperback / eBook

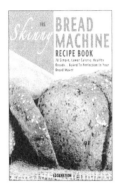

THE SKINNY BREAD MACHINE RECIPE BOOK

70 Simple, Lower Calorie, Healthy Breads...Baked To Perfection In Your Bread Maker.

Paperback / eBook

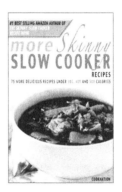

MORE SKINNY SLOW COOKER RECIPES

75 More Delicious Recipes Under 300, 400 & 500 Calories.

Paperback / eBook

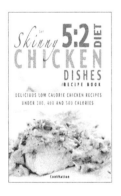

THE SKINNY 5:2 DIET CHICKEN DISHES RECIPE BOOK

Delicious Low Calorie Chicken Dishes Under 300, 400 & 500 Calories.

Paperback / eBook

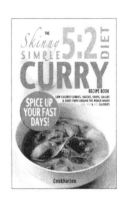

THE SKINNY 5:2 CURRY RECIPE BOOK

Spice Up Your Fast Days With Simple Low Calorie Curries, Snacks, Soups, Salads & Sides Under 200, 300 & 400 Calories.

Paperback / eBook

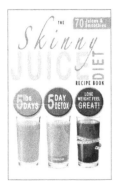

THE SKINNY JUICE DIET RECIPE BOOK

5lbs, 5 Days. The Ultimate Kick- Start Diet and Detox Plan to Lose Weight & Feel Great!

Paperback / eBook

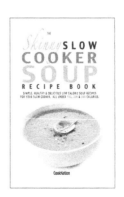

THE SKINNY SLOW COOKER SOUP RECIPE BOOK

Simple, Healthy & Delicious Low Calorie Soup Recipes For Your Slow Cooker. All Under 100, 200 & 300 Calories.

Paperback / eBook

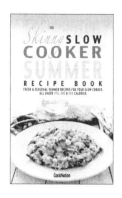

THE SKINNY SLOW COOKER SUMMER RECIPE BOOK

Fresh & Seasonal Summer Recipes For Your Slow Cooker. All Under 300, 400 And 500 Calories.

Paperback / eBook

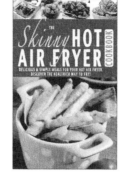

THE SKINNY HOT AIR FRYER COOKBOOK

Delicious & Simple Meals For Your Hot Air Fryer: Discover The Healthier Way To Fry.

Paperback / eBook

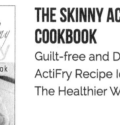

THE SKINNY ACTIFRY COOKBOOK

Guilt-free and Delicious ActiFry Recipe Ideas: Discover The Healthier Way to Fry!

Paperback / eBook

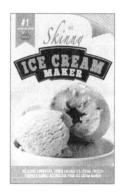

THE SKINNY ICE CREAM MAKER

Delicious Lower Fat, Lower Calorie Ice Cream, Frozen Yogurt & Sorbet Recipes For Your Ice Cream Maker.

Paperback / eBook

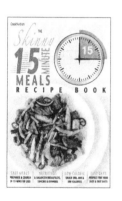

THE SKINNY 15 MINUTE MEALS RECIPE BOOK

Delicious, Nutritious & Super-Fast Meals in 15 Minutes Or Less. All Under 300, 400 & 500 Calories.

Paperback / eBook

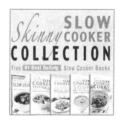

THE SKINNY SLOW COOKER COLLECTION

5 Fantastic Books of Delicious, Diet-friendly Skinny Slow Cooker Recipes: ALL Under 200, 300, 400 & 500 Calories! **eBook**

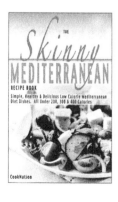

THE SKINNY MEDITERRANEAN RECIPE BOOK

Simple, Healthy & Delicious Low Calorie Mediterranean Diet Dishes. All Under 200, 300 & 400 Calories.

Paperback / eBook

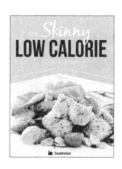

THE SKINNY LOW CALORIE RECIPE BOOK

Great Tasting, Simple & Healthy Meals Under 300, 400 & 500 Calories. Perfect For Any Calorie Controlled Diet.

Paperback / eBook

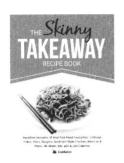

THE SKINNY TAKEAWAY RECIPE BOOK

Healthier Versions Of Your Fast Food Favourites: All Under 300, 400 & 500 Calories.

Paperback / eBook

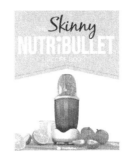

THE SKINNY NUTRIBULLET RECIPE BOOK

80+ Delicious & Nutritious Healthy Smoothie Recipes. Burn Fat, Lose Weight and Feel Great!

Paperback / eBook

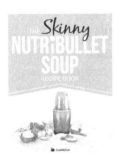

THE SKINNY NUTRIBULLET SOUP RECIPE BOOK

Delicious, Quick & Easy, Single Serving Soups & Pasta Sauces For Your Nutribullet. All Under 100, 200, 300 & 400 Calories!

Paperback / eBook

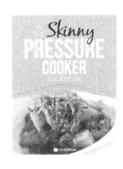

THE SKINNY PRESSURE COOKER COOKBOOK

USA ONLY
Low Calorie, Healthy & Delicious Meals, Sides & Desserts. All Under 300, 400 & 500 Calories.

Paperback / eBook

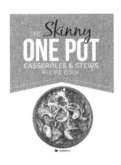

THE SKINNY ONE-POT RECIPE BOOK

Simple & Delicious, One-Pot Meals. All Under 300, 400 & 500 Calories

Paperback / eBook

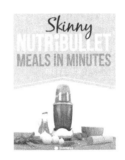

THE SKINNY NUTRIBULLET MEALS IN MINUTES RECIPE BOOK

Quick & Easy, Single Serving Suppers, Snacks, Sauces, Salad Dressings & More Using Your Nutribullet. All Under 300, 400 & 500 Calories

Paperback / eBook

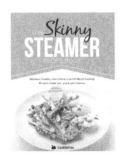

THE SKINNY STEAMER RECIPE BOOK

Healthy, Low Calorie, Low Fat Steam Cooking Recipes Under 300, 400 & 500 Calories.

Paperback / eBook

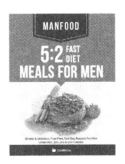

MANFOOD: 5:2 FAST DIET MEALS FOR MEN

Simple & Delicious, Fuss Free, Fast Day Recipes For Men Under 200, 300, 400 & 500 Calories.

Paperback / eBook

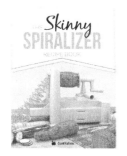

THE SKINNY SPIRALIZER RECIPE BOOK

Delicious Spiralizer Inspired Low Calorie Recipes For One. All Under 200, 300, 400 & 500 Calories

Paperback / eBook

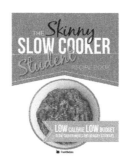

THE SKINNY SLOW COOKER STUDENT RECIPE BOOK

Delicious, Simple, Low Calorie, Low Budget, Slow Cooker Meals For Hungry Students. All Under 300, 400 & 500 Calories

Paperback / eBook

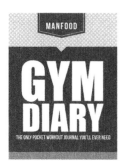

MANFOOD: GYM DIARY:

The Only Pocket Workout Journal You'll Ever Need

Paperback / eBook

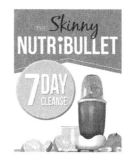

THE SKINNY NUTRIBULLET 7 DAY CLEANSE

Calorie Counted Cleanse & Detox Plan: Smoothies, Soups & Meals to Lose Weight & Feel Great Fast. Real Food. Real Results

Paperback / eBook

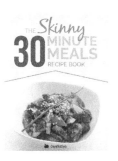

THE SKINNY 30 MINUTE MEALS RECIPE BOOK

Great Food, Easy Recipes, Prepared & Cooked In 30 Minutes Or Less. All Under 300, 400 & 500 Calories

Paperback / eBook

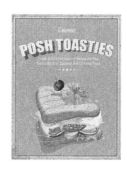

POSH TOASTIES

Simple & Delicious Gourmet Recipes For Your Toastie Machine, Sandwich Grill Or Panini Press

Paperback / eBook

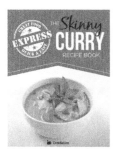

THE SKINNY EXPRESS CURRY RECIPE BOOK

Quick & Easy Authentic Low Fat Indian Dishes Under 300, 400 & 500 Calories

Paperback / eBook

Lightning Source UK Ltd.
Milton Keynes UK
UKOW07f0942260515

252281UK00001B/3/P